IV NAD For Treating Drug Addictions

A Holistic Approach for Brain Restoration and Recovering Physical & Mental Health

By Dr. Alexander Haskell, ND

Copyright © 2018 by Dr. Alexander Haskell, ND

All rights reserved.

ISBN-13: 978-1719184373
ISBN-10: 1719184372

Table of Contents

SECTION I 1

  THE USE OF IV NAD 3
    Collateral Damage 4
    Symptoms Are the Messenger 4
    Mitochondrial Dysfunction 5
    NAD to the Rescue 6
    Pathogens & Cellular Dysfunction 6
  NAD & MITOCHONDRIAL FUNCTION 9
    Mitochondrial Dysfunction 9
    Causes & Solutions for Mitochondrial Dysfunction 10
    NAD & The Krebs Cycle 11
  JOURNEY OF DRUG RESIDUES 15
    From the Lymph into the Bloodstream 17
    Through the Liver, Kidneys & Gall Bladder 17
    Small & Large Intestines 19
    Fat Cells, Primary Storage Site for Residues 20
    A Case in Point 21
        Thyroid Hormones 23
        Blood Sugar 23
        Fats 25
        Vitamin D 26
        Female Hormones 26
        Dark-field Microscope 27

SECTION II 29

  BASIC NATUROPATHIC PRINCIPLES 31
    Symptoms Are the Messenger 32
    The Three Primary Causes of Chronic Illness 33
        Nutritional Deficiencies 33
        Environmental Toxins 36
        Pathogens 37
  ONE ANALOGY OF DRUG SIDE-EFFECTS 39
    Stop Filling the Bowl 40
    Empty the Bowl 41
    Tipping the Scales 41
  PURIFICATION THERAPIES FOR RECOVERY 45

Lymphatic Hydrotherapy 45
    The Procedure 46
Colon Hydrotherapy 48
    The Procedure 49
Saunas to the Rescue 50
    The Benefits of Sauna 50
    The Sauna Experience 51
    Walk-in Dry Sauna 51
The Bemer 52
Photon Sound Beam 53
LIST OF THERAPIES 55
Nutritional IVs 56
IVs for Pathogens 57
Zotzmann 10-Pass Hyperbaric Ozone Therapy 58
UBI or Bio-Photonic Therapy 59
High-Dose Vitamin C 60

SECTION III 61

COMPREHENSIVE TESTING TO ASSESS UNDERLYING CAUSES 63
LabCorp of America 63
DHA Laboratory 64
Cell Science Systems Lab 64
Labrix 65
Dark-field Microscope 65
Electrodermal Screening 66

SECTION IV 69

SUMMARY & HIGHLIGHTS 71

SECTION V 73

BECOMING A CLIENT 75
Clients in Utah 75
Long Distance Clients 78
CONTACT INFORMATION 85

SECTION I

The Use of IV NAD

We have been using intravenous NAD for about eight years, primarily for people wanting to discontinue their prescription due to side-effects, who have tried to withdraw, but cannot.

Overall, NAD has been successful, with some results being miraculous while others rather mediocre.

In the past, a moderate percentage of clients had to return for additional IVs of NAD because of a recurrence of their symptoms, even though they had abstained from taking any medication or drugs.

About six months ago, we decided to stop using IV NAD as a stand-alone therapy, because we realized it did not address other causes for why people were experiencing physical and mental symptoms.

Sure, people were definitely suffering from drug side-effects but there were other reasons as well.

The simplistic belief that health issues, due to drugs and other causes, will be resolved by the use of NAD has been unfortunately fostered by quick-fix, panacea promising clinics offering this therapy.

Recovering physical and mental health just isn't that simple.

Why?

Collateral Damage

First, every drug will cause some degree of damage to the cells of our body.

These must be repaired.

Every physician knows that almost all drugs must be carefully prescribed.

An overdose can lead to severe consequences, even death.

We can therefore consider most drugs, because they are synthesized and foreign to the body, to be toxic or poisonous.

Even when we take a pharmaceutical at the prescribed dosage, we are still taking in a little bit of poison every day, which leads to some degree of harm at the cellular level.

In some cases, this damage may be irreparable, but in many, it can be repaired.

This repair must focus on cellular membranes, intercellular organelles and DNA.

NAD is a godsend for clearing drug and environmental toxins from inside our cells, but NAD, by itself, will not repair.

NAD does help to activate the healing mechanisms of the cell, but the nutrients, proteins and lipids needed by the cell for repair must be provided.

Symptoms Are the Messenger

Second, for the most part, a person is given a prescription because they presented with symptoms to their physician.

Most of the time, this prescription does not address or resolve the reasons or causes for why the person had symptoms in the first place.

A prescription may help reduce symptoms but it does not

address the causes.

The symptoms may improve from the prescription, but the causes remain.

For chronic conditions, a prescription is usually not a cure, in the true sense of the word.

Symptoms usually subside on the prescription, but if the prescription is stopped, the symptoms will return, so it is not a cure.

What are symptoms?

Symptoms are the means by which our body communicates to us that something is not right, and it is the duty of the clinician to investigate these symptoms, not to simply label them and to prescribe a medication to silence them.

What I am saying here, is this.

The symptoms a person associates with the side-effects of a drug are very likely the combination of the drug *and* the symptoms experienced before receiving the prescription.

Most of the time, these other causes for symptoms will not be addressed or improved with NAD.

Mitochondrial Dysfunction

Third, the primary reason for why drugs lead to side-effects is because the effect their residues have upon the inner workings of our cells.

The action of drugs only happens on the cellular level.

Water soluble drugs have their primary effect upon cellular membrane receptors, while the action of lipid-soluble drugs occurs inside of cells.

Normally, these intercellular drug residues are transported outside our cells across the cell's membrane.

This excretion is considered an 'active' transport, meaning it requires energy (ATP), energy produced by organelles inside the cell, called mitochondria.

After some time of ingesting a drug, more and more intercellular drug begin to negatively affect the activity of these mitochondria.

Eventually, the production of energy declines and the cell becomes overwhelmed by these residues, and symptoms, or side-effects, become more severe.

We now have symptoms due to mitochondrial dysfunction, with the root cause being drug residues.

This becomes a vicious downward spiral.

We must find a way to feed our mitochondria in order to increase energy production.

NAD to the Rescue

One of the primary actions of NAD is to stimulate mitochondria to produce more ATP, and thus help to transport drug resides across cell membranes and out of the cell.

But mitochondria require many other nutrients to produce ATP, and if these nutrients remain deficient, once the series of IV NAD is complete, very slowly but surely, the production of ATP will decline, and symptoms will return.

Pathogens & Cellular Dysfunction

Fourth, I mentioned the need to address underlying causes of symptoms besides drug residues, and, in our experience, many of our clients present with chronic, low-grade, systemic infections.

These can be bacterial, viral and mold, and these are systemic, meaning they are circulating in the blood throughout the body.

These living organisms rob us of nutrients and also excrete their toxic waste products referred to as biotoxins or exotoxins.

Many people are unable to completely clear these molecular toxins, giving rise to a wide variety of physical and mental symptoms.

These biotoxins find their way inside cells, and, just like drugs, can be another reason for developing mitochondrial dysfunction.

NAD, since it stimulates mitochondria to produce ATP, will help to clear this waste from within our cells.

BUT, if these blood pathogens are not reduced using various oxidative therapies, then any benefits from the IV NAD will slowly decline as these biotoxins continue to enter cells.

Next, it best to explain how NAD works along with a few complications that may arise from NAD.

NAD & Mitochondrial Function

Let's dive into the interior of a cell to understand why NAD is the most effective means of detoxification and the recovery of cellular health.

On the physical plane we are composed of over 40 trillion cells, and your overall health is a reflection of the sum total function of all these cells.

Therefore, we could say that if your cells are functioning optimally, then you would be healthy and symptom free.

But if their function declines, then symptoms will appear.

Mitochondrial Dysfunction

Inside every cell, except for red blood cells, are small organelles called mitochondria.

The most important activity of these organelles is to generate energy (ATP) which drives the cell's function.

If the mitochondria's production of ATP declines, then the function of that cell also declines.

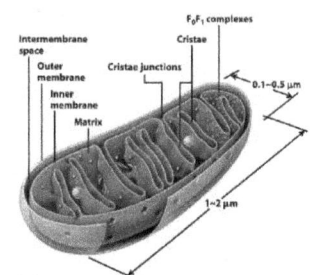

If it's a thyroid cell, then the production of thyroid hormones declines and the person experiences hypothyroid symptoms such as fatigue and depression.

If it's a cell that secretes serotonin, then its' production declines and the person may experience depression and insomnia.

As far as recovery and the resurrection of health, the objective must then be to increase mitochondrial function to receive and experience all the benefits of increased energy.

Causes & Solutions for Mitochondrial Dysfunction

Mitochondria need specific nutrients to function optimally, to make plenty of ATP, and nutritional deficiencies are one cause of lowered mitochondrial function.

These nutrients include most of the B vitamins, various trace minerals, amino acids and anti-oxidants. Specific foods rich in phytonutrients are essential.

The second cause of mitochondrial dysfunction is the accumulation of toxic residues within the cell, from synthetic chemicals (drugs), many environmental insults, and biotoxins excreted by pathogens.

Mitochondrial dysfunction caused by drugs is the reason we experience side-effects.

When we stop a drug, we still experience these same symptoms of side-effects because we still have drug residues inside cells which continue to promote mitochondrial dysfunction.

Not until we feed our mitochondria through nutrition and specific supplements, as well as NAD, will we ever reduce side-effects and recover our health.

NAD & The Krebs Cycle

It is bewildering how much knowledge we have about the intricacies of how we function.

We have turned our search from the stellar heavens towards the inner constellations of the human being.

We will never fathom the miraculous intelligence which motivates the intricate activity, cooperation and communication existing within a single cell.

Since we wish to understand the effects of NAD, we must know something about the inner workings of an organelle with the cell called the mitochondria.

On average, their length is about two microns. If we lay 50,000 mitochondria end to end, the length is about two inches.

Within the mitochondria, energy is produced in what's termed the Krebs Cycle.

On the next page is a diagram of this cycle, showing the basic nutrients required for optimal mitochondrial function, as well as NAD.

I've placed plus signs next to the nutrients and large arrows next to NAD. The rectangular box contains other essential nutrients.

Krebs Cycle Nutrients

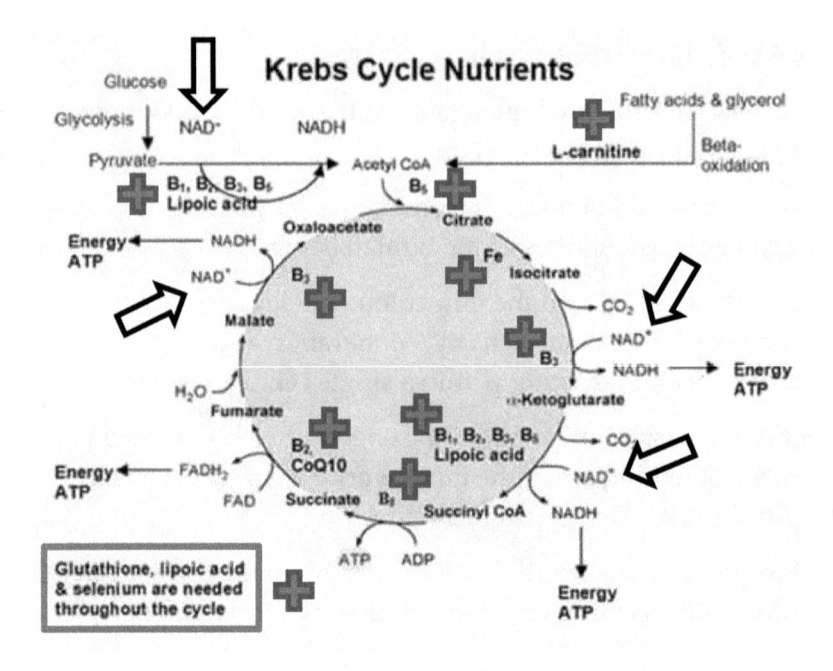

(Diagram showing the Krebs cycle with nutrients: Glucose → Glycolysis (NAD⁺ → NADH) → Pyruvate → Acetyl CoA (with B₁, B₂, B₃, B₅, Lipoic acid); Fatty acids & glycerol → L-carnitine → Beta-oxidation → Acetyl CoA (B₅); Citrate → Isocitrate (Fe) → α-Ketoglutarate (B₃) → Succinyl CoA (B₁, B₂, B₃, B₅, Lipoic acid) → Succinate (B₃) → Fumarate (B₂, CoQ10) → Malate (B₃) → Oxaloacetate (B₃); with NAD⁺/NADH, FAD/FADH₂, ATP/ADP, CO₂, H₂O producing Energy ATP. Glutathione, lipoic acid & selenium are needed throughout the cycle.)

This cycle depicts ATP production in a clockwise fashion.

Notice that NAD becomes NADH which results in energy or ATP.

To produce the maximum amount of ATP, this cycle must be completed, and if any nutrients are missing, then the full cycle of ATP production is compromised.

So this is the level at which IV NAD is working, to accelerate and to complete this cycle.

Obviously, you can see how important NAD is, but you must also admit that if these other nutrients are lacking, then the full benefits of NAD will never occur.

Remember, the excretion of drug residues and other toxins from within the cell is an active transport requiring ATP.

The benefits of NAD are two-fold; improving the function of

cells by accelerating the output of ATP and increasing the excretion of drug residues.

All this leads to the reduction of symptoms, but, still, this is not enough.

JOURNEY OF DRUG RESIDUES

Let us now take a journey, of a drug residue which has just been excreted from a cell.

The first fluid it enters is lymph.

Lymph bathes every cell of the body, it passively transports nutrients absorbed from the intestines and hormones secreted by various glands, and carries away metabolic waste produced by our cells.

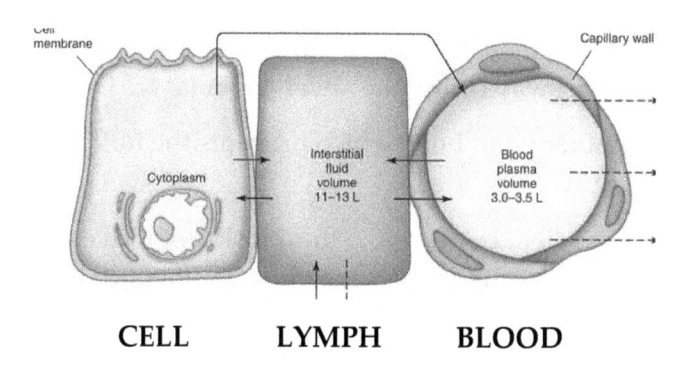

CELL   LYMPH   BLOOD

The flow of lymph is somewhat dependent upon our physical activity, since the contraction and relaxation of the muscles surrounding lymph vessels helps to pump or move lymph fluid.

Lymph fluid slowly empties or drains into our bloodstream through ducts or ports just under our right and left clavicle bones.

The lymph system is a pathway which is vital for detoxification, yet seldom is this system recognized in medicine as being important.

Problems with NAD detoxification arise when a person's lymph system is more like a swamp than a river.

So what about this drug residue which has just arrived in this lymph swamp and just sits there, unable to flow into the bloodstream?

The result is that the person feels just awful, with various ill symptoms, what is referred to as a Herx reaction.

In some people with severe lymph stasis, their symptoms may become so extreme that they cannot continue with NAD.

This is very unfortunate because this aggravation may last for days, weeks or months.

Now we understand how important lymphatic drainage is for certain people, way before they ever begin IV NAD.

There's another point here, which prevents the full benefits of NAD therapy.

There is a gradient between the fluid inside of the cell and the fluid outside the cell (lymph), meaning a difference in the concentration (osmolarity) of these fluids.

When the lymph is congested, and cells are in the process of excreting toxins, there becomes a point when residues can no longer be excreted.

In this case, when a person has finished their course of NAD and feels somewhat better, it won't be long before those chemical residues in the lymph will reenter the cells once again.

But let's say the lymph is moving like a stream and this drug residue finds its way into the bloodstream.

From the Lymph into the Bloodstream

This drug residue, whether it passes through the right or left thoracic duct, enters the subclavian (below the clavicle) vein which leads directly to the heart.

Heart tissue is very sensitive to chemicals and toxins, with the typical reaction being increased heart rate.

If someone has cardiac issues, they may require support before and during IV NAD.

Typical suggestions are Coenzyme Q10, Gingko biloba, magnesium, potassium and the herb Hawthorne.

After traveling through the right chambers of the heart, this residue travels to and through the lungs, back to the left chambers of the heart, and then exits into the arteries.

Now there are several possibilities of where this residue can travel.

- Through the hepatic artery to the liver
- Through the renal artery to the kidneys
- Through any tissue via capillaries, the smallest blood vessels
- From the capillaries through the hepatic portal vein and into the liver

Through the Liver, Kidneys & Gall Bladder

The liver may metabolize this drug residue in two ways.

Since most of the drugs we are dealing with are fat-soluble, the liver can either make it a water-soluble residue or filter it and send it to the gall bladder.

The water-soluble form is filtered and excreted through the kidneys.

Rarely have we seen anyone with compromised kidney function, but in a few cases, both the Physical Energetics product, Solidago, and fresh, organic beet and celery juice have helped.

Liver issues are extremely common because of the accumulation of drug residues inside liver cells which has led to mitochondrial dysfunction, so the fat soluble drug residue can cause some issues.

But NAD is great for improving liver function by increasing ATP production within liver cells.

The supplement Mitocore is designed to provide all the nutrients needed by mitochondria, but liver cell mitochondria have high requirements for Alpha Lipoic Acid, Glutathione and Inositol.

The gall bladder, just under the liver, is very often an issue because of the accumulation of fat soluble waste products, chemicals and drug residues.

During IV NAD, a common complaint is nausea, and this is typically a symptom of gall bladder congestion.

Way before a person starts IV NAD, they must begin supporting liver function and draining the gall bladder.

There is no reason to suffer unnecessarily and the faster we can help the body to excrete these residues and prevent them from hanging out in tissues and fluids, the better the long-term outcome of IV NAD will be.

For gall bladder drainage, the most important herb is

artichoke. There's a great formula from Physica called Dandi Intrinsic which contains artichoke, milk thistle, dandelion and four other herbs.

So let's assume this little drug residue has made its way through the lymph, blood, liver and gall bladder, and has now passed into the duodenum portion of the upper small intestines.

Small & Large Intestines

It seems like everyone these days has some type of gut issue, likely due to a combination of poor digestion, gall bladder issues, the overuse of antibiotics, bacterial overgrowth, fungus, food allergies, leaky gut, inflammation or Irritable Bowel Syndrome, and parasites.

Whew…!

With NAD, how do you think the gut is going to react when we start dumping drug residues into this mix?

Dealing with gut issues before starting IV NAD is absolutely necessary.

And when people begin improving the health of their gut, many experience a reduction of their symptoms, symptoms they had associated with the side-effects of their drug(s).

They feel very encouraged when they start feeling better without having even started the IV NAD.

There are many ways to deal with these gut issues and the approach depends upon what's going on.

- **Digestive Issues:** Various digestive enzymes
- **Gall Bladder:** Bile salts, concentrated beet extract and artichoke extract (Dandi)
- **Bacteria:** Probiotics, olive leaf extract, Biocidin,

Tanalbit and Berberine
- **Fungus:** Probiotics, Caprylic acid, and many others
- **Food Allergies:** Digestive enzymes, hypoallergenic diet
- **Leaky Gut:** L-Glutamine and Aloe Vera, rich in mucopolysaccharides
- **Parasites:** Para 1, Albendazole, Ivermectin, etc.

Most of the time, we recommend dietary changes which help to correct many of the conditions listed above.

And when drug residues enter the intestines and must then travel about 20 to 25 feet before they are evacuated, we must ensure these residues will not be assimilated through the gut lining to reenter the lymph and blood.

Therefore, using binders before and during the NAD is recommended.

- Charcoal from organic coconut
- PectaSol

If constipation is an issue, this must be resolved before starting IV NAD.

- High dose magnesium
- High dose buffered vitamin C to bowel tolerance
- Nat Colon CLR from Physica Energetics

Fat Cells, Primary Storage Site for Residues

We've talked about how NAD detoxifies drug residues from cells by increasing mitochondrial function.

But some cells, like fat cells, have only a few mitochondria, so the benefits of NAD will be less in these cells.

It turns out that fat cells are the primary site where the body loves to compartmentalize both drug residues and environmental toxins.

The body's wisdom does everything it can to protect vital tissues like our reproductive organs and our brain and neurological system.

So it chooses fat cells, maybe our least important cells, to shunt these residues into.

This, of course, causes the same issue with mitochondrial dysfunction, with a lowered metabolic rate or activity of these cells.

This may be another reason why it is so challenging for many people to lose weight, since the excretion of fat from fat cells is compromised.

Besides excreting toxins from fat cells into the lymph, there is another pathway of detoxification that is easier and with immediate benefits, and this is through the skin.

Saunas are key.

Just below the skin lies the subdermal fat layer, and toxins can exit these fat cells through the pores in the skin when we perspire.

We always encourage clients to begin saunas immediately and to use our sauna every day during the IV NAD.

A Case in Point

To understand this journey in a practical sense, here's a case of a woman in her late 30s who wanted NAD because of health issues she felt related to Citalopram (Celexa), an SSRI, prescribed by her physician a year ago for depression.

At that time, the physician told her that all her labs were

normal and said her condition was rooted in a psychological issue.

For the first six months she had felt somewhat better but then side-effects began to appear;

- Mild weight gain
- Declining interest in sex
- Mild nausea at times
- Her insomnia had become worse
- Some drowsiness & fatigue

She had returned to her physician with these complaints, who wanted to 'try' a different medication, but when she read the possible side-effects, she declined.

She felt trapped because when she tried to tapper, her symptoms became even worse and her depression returned with greater severity.

She worked on her nutrition and somehow found the energy to exercise. She joined a yoga class and made a greater effort to be with friends.

All the above helped but she felt desperate.

When we met she reviewed her lifestyle and symptoms.

She had a history of eating poorly, of being on a low-caloric, low-fat diet because she wanted to lose weight.

She had issues with digestion and was likely not assimilating nutrients from her gut.

Therefore, all her cells were undernourished, and I made the assumption that some of her symptoms were due to lowered mitochondrial function.

With occasional nausea and tenderness over her liver and gall bladder, there was likely an issue with detoxification and the inability to efficiently clear toxins.

She had mild pitting edema or swelling, so her lymph system was not flowing freely.

She suffered from constipation.

In a case like this, where do we start?

Do we simply begin the IVs of NAD?

Hell no!

First, we must know what's going on with her biochemistry and hormones, which meant getting some labs.

Here are the highlights.

Thyroid Hormones

Her thyroid hormones (*TSH, T4, Free T4, Free T3 and thyroid TPO & TGA antibodies*) were within the normal lab range but two of them, one being most important (*Free T3*), was right at the bottom end of the range.

A physician would usually interpret these results as 'normal' and pass over them, but I felt her suboptimal levels were contributing to her fatigue and depression.

I offered her the diagnosis of 'suboptimal hypothyroidism.'

We prescribed a low dose of thyroid medication and a couple of trace minerals to 'feed' her thyroid cells.

Blood Sugar

Besides various nutrients, our cells require two things, oxygen and glucose; no oxygen and we die, no glucose and we slip into a coma.

Could some of her symptoms be due to inadequate glucose, or that glucose was not getting into her cells?

A fasting glucose blood test tells us the resting blood sugar after not eating for 12 hours, though it does not tell us what happens to blood sugar before and between meals.

Her fasting glucose result was a little low at 72, still within the reference range but not optimal, being 85 to 90.

Another lab test called glycosylated hemoglobin (HA1c) measures the glucose on the hemoglobin protein of red blood cells, and since the life span of a red cell is three months, this result tells us her average blood sugar over the last 90 days.

Her HA1c was 4.5, and if we calculate this to the same units as glucose (*mg/dl*), her average blood glucose was 83.

This meant that, not only was her fasting glucose suboptimal, but that she was frequently dipping into low blood sugar or hypoglycemia.

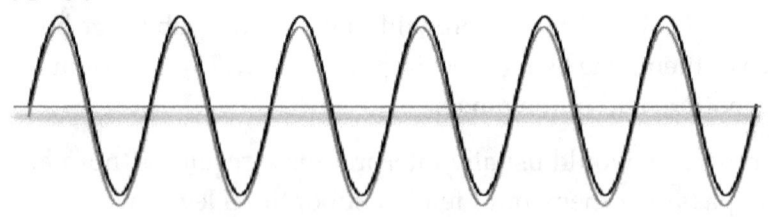

So now we had another cause for her symptoms, that the cells of her body and brain were under-functioning because they weren't getting enough glucose when she slipped into hypoglycemia.

The low-caloric, low-fat diet she'd been following for the last 10 years certainly wasn't helping.

Our nutritionist designed a menu with her, recommending more calories based upon her weight, and increasing her protein and fat intake.

Fats

This brings us to another lab test that might explain why she was experiencing symptoms.

Because of her diet, I suspected a nutrient deficiency that relates to her insomnia, low blood sugar, pain (she had hip pain), fatigue, depression and many others.

All these issues can be due to low levels of two hormones, cortisol and progesterone.

These two hormones, plus several others, are steroid hormones and the glands that make them require a specific nutrient.

What's this vital nutrient these glands require?

Cholesterol.

Low levels of this nutrient will lead to inadequate or suboptimal production of these steroid hormones.

Her lab result for cholesterol was 121, with an optimal being around 185.

Here was another cause for her symptoms.

She recalled her doctor had said her cholesterol was fantastic, that seldom had he seen anyone with this low of a cholesterol unless they had been taking a lipid lowering drug.

'Keep up what you're eating, and you'll never die of a heart attack.'

Well, that may be true, but what about quality of life and all the physical and mental symptoms related to low cholesterol and low steroid hormones?

Once this woman understood the necessity of cholesterol, and that it wasn't fats that would make her fat, but rather sugars and refined starches, it was an easy shift for her to follow our recommendations.

Vitamin D

Because this woman was very concerned with ageing and wrinkles, she never went outdoors in the sun for long unless she applied sunscreen.

Her lab result for vitamin D was 28 with an optimal level for a female being 60-70.

Low levels of vitamin D can cause depression, fatigue, and muscle aches and pains.

She was put on 10,000 units a day, of an emulsified form for easy assimilation.

Female Hormones

Upon more detailed questioning, she mentioned that her poor sleep, now and before the prescription, was worse the week before her periods.

She also had minor headaches during this premenstrual time.

We ran saliva hormone testing for one of the estrogens (estradiol) and progesterone.

The results showed a pretty severe progesterone deficiency, maybe due to her low cholesterol, and even though her estradiol was fine, she had estrogen dominance, a calculated ratio between her estradiol and progesterone.

The easiest, quickest and most effective way to correct this is to take oral bioidentical progesterone, about 150mgs before bed.

By the way, after just three nights, her sleep had greatly improved.

Dark-field Microscope

We viewed a tiny drop of her blood (finger stick) under a dark-field microscope to see if any bacteria, signs of viral issues or mold showed up.

All was clear except for some mold.

We didn't think this was much of an issue compared with the other lab results, yet because she was sensitive to odors and fragrances, we recommended a homeopathic remedy to reduce her sensitivity and to get her home checked for mold using a test kit from moldcheck.com.

We ran many other labs but the above were the abnormal ones.

We started with supplementation, thyroid hormones, nutritional guidelines, vitamin D, oral progesterone and a few products to improve her liver function and gut health.

During the next two weeks we also started her on some purification therapies including saunas and lymphatic drainage.

Even before starting IV NAD, she was feeling much better.

So we recommended tapering her prescription and to begin the 10 days of IV NAD.

She came out of the 10-Day NAD IV Program feeling extremely well.

In the beginning, here were the concerns we had to consider.

If we had initially used IV NAD to stimulate her mitochondria in order to excrete drug residues from her cells, she would have felt much worse since they would have entered her stagnant lymph system.

With her lymph being one site for toxins which she had accumulated over her life, if we began draining her lymph fluid, these toxins would have travelled into her blood and placed a burden on her liver which was already taxed.

If her liver began to filter and spill more toxins into her intestines, because of her constipation, she'd feel worse.

So with purification (*emptying the bowl*) we need to begin downstream from cellular detoxification and, in her case, we focused on her colon.

Within a few days of getting her bowels to move, we started lymphatic drainage and supplements to support her liver and gall bladder.

We also started to feed her mitochondrial, using supplements like Mitocore and some intravenous nutrients.

Then, after the two weeks and being off her medication, we started intravenous NAD and some IV antioxidants to neutralize free radicals.

Throughout this time, we encouraged saunas for detoxification through the skin.

I hope I have explained the importance of simultaneously opening the pathways of detoxification, of providing various nutrients and the need for purification therapies, in conjunction with the use of IV NAD.

The next section reviews some principle of health and the reasons or causes of symptoms and illness.

It is not necessarily about NAD but how we must address underlying issues first, to maximize the benefits of NAD.

SECTION II

Basic Naturopathic Principles

Illness does not arrive like a thief in the night but gradually and silently seeps into our life.

There must be reasons for this.

There must be causes!

I believe that under utopian conditions (agricultural, environmental, social, financial & political) we should be able to live our lives in perfect health.

Yet this ideal is seldom the case and we naively call upon our highly advanced, technologically sophisticated system of medicine for the cure.

But the system does not take into consideration the multiple causes of chronic disease. This is in part due to the pharmaceutical industry's influence upon the education of physicians and this industry's lack of concern for addressing causes.

Why is it that so many known chemical carcinogens are dismissed by our FDA and EPA as being harmless, though research has proven the opposite to be true?

How long will we continue to entrust our health to our government and for-profit corporations?

How has our society become so naïve about the long-term potential side-effects of synthetic drugs?

We have strayed far from the art of medicine, which historically considered symptoms as the body's struggle to bring itself back into balance and regulation.

But many people are seeking the light, realizing that drugs are not the answer.

Symptoms Are the Messenger

Let's be clear about physical and mental symptoms, their origin and what they truly mean.

I strongly believe that everyone possesses the capacity to heal, and I refer to this capacity as an innate wisdom which is superior in knowledge to the most enlightened physician.

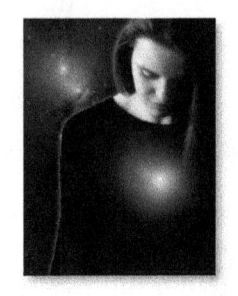

I recall the subject of physiology in pre-med with the 1st chapter being devoted to homeostasis, the ability of the body (innate wisdom) to maintain the biochemical and hormonal balance of hundreds if not thousands of mechanisms within a healthy range.

I was extremely fortunate to have a professor who continued to remind us of this miraculous capacity, that the body possesses this incomprehensible ability to monitor, regulate and correct any deviation from 'normal.'

Over the years I've come to understand more deeply how this wisdom has been actively and untiringly engaged in maintaining this balance ever since the moment of conception, day in and day out, until this present moment in time.

Describing it as miraculous is an understatement.

This means we each possess our own inner physician which has the ability to restore and maintain our health, while communicating to us through the language of physical and mental symptoms.

These symptoms can appear in an acute situation or the milder onset of chronic symptoms such as aches and pains, dizziness, fatigue, headaches or digestive issues.

These symptoms communicate to us that something is not right, that we need to investigate the underlying reasons for them, rather than immediately turning to some medication for relief.

I believe this is the most important mindset for anyone trying to recover their health.

There are always reasons, always causes for why we experience unpleasant symptoms.

And with this, we begin to nurture an attitude, that symptoms are the voice of our innate physician attempting to get our attention, and to bring us back into balance.

Through our attentiveness and appreciation for this wisdom within, we can then participate in assisting this intelligence during the process of recovery and regulation.

The Three Primary Causes of Chronic Illness

Nutritional Deficiencies

So here are some thoughts to consider around the causes of illness.

Over 2,000 years ago, the Father of Medicine, Hippocrates, believed chronic ailments had two primary causes.

The 1st cause is nutritional deficiencies.

This makes common sense.

If our cells do not receive the nutrients they require to function optimally, then naturally our physical and mental health will decline.

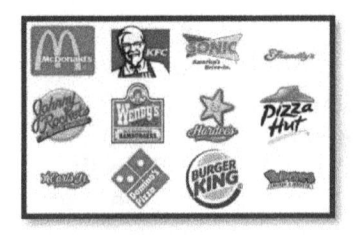

For many, this state of semi-starvation manifests in a wide variety of symptoms, yet seldom do we or our physicians consider our symptoms being partly due to nutrient deficiencies.

Then there was Dr. Weston Price, DDS, who studied the effects of food upon health and disease.

One of the most elegant nutritional research studies was performed by Dr. Price, and supports the first cause of illness being nutritional deficiencies.

While practicing dentistry during the late 1800s and early 1900s, Price was curious as to why children presented with far more dental issues than their parents.

His practice was during the time of advancing technologies in the processing and manufacturing of foods from companies like Kellogg's and Nabisco.

Price wondered if these dental changes might be due to the introduction and consumption of these less nutritious, industrialized foods.

He decided to visit isolated regions of the world where people's nutrition was still restricted to locally grown foods.

Dr. Price and his wife traveled to the Swiss Alps, the coast of

Scotland, Eskimo and Indian tribes in Canada, the aborigines of Australia, the Maoris of New Zealand, the Amazonian Indians and the tribesmen in Africa.

At that time, these indigenous people lived in remote locations far from the influence of 'Western' foods and environmental toxins.

Price kept immaculate and journalistic style notes accompanied by photographs to illustrate his findings.

Price found that in each group every individual exhibited both dental and physical health.

Infirmities and disease were for the most part absent.

Tooth decay was extremely rare and dental crowding was nonexistent.

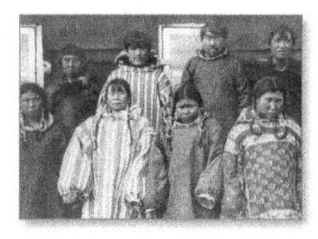

Over many decades Price returned to these communities to witness increased dental decay and a variety of chronic illnesses with the only variable being food stuffs imported by traders and missionaries.

These new foods were primarily white sugar, refined grains, canned foods, pasteurized milk and 'devitalized' fats and oils.

These foods were not only less wholesome and nutrient deficient than local foods but also displaced the consumption of foods normally eaten by these people.

If you have an interest in learning more about Dr. Price to understand how our 'modern' foods are at the root of our epidemic in chronic illness, pick up a copy of *Nutrition & Physical Degeneration*.

Environmental Toxins

Hippocrates stated the 2nd cause of degenerative disease was toxins and many physicians over the centuries have also realized the negative impact environmental chemicals have upon health.

It seems obvious that when these foreign toxins enter our bodies in small yet persistent amounts, over time the body will express subtle symptoms which become progressively worse.

This is why a physician must investigate a client's living, working and surrounding environments, hobbies and gardening activities, food and water sources, mold exposure and their chronological chemical history of exposure.

Just because a person's symptoms developed recently, it's quite possible that a seed was planted decades before.

It is obviously futile to treat present symptoms without considering why, and the circumstances around which they developed.

So if our innate physician is communicating to us through physical and mental symptoms, how do we go about correcting the possible causes?

With toxins, the 1st step is avoidance, to remove the cause or causes in order to reduce our exposure.

The 2nd is to assist our innate wisdom through purification therapies.

How to do this will be discussed later.

But there are other causes in addition to nutritional deficiencies and environmental toxins which other clinicians since Hippocrates have recognized as causative.

Pathogens

Louis Pasteur ushered in the germ theory, that micro-organisms were the cause of acute and chronic illness.

This is true, but another 19th century French scientist, Claude Bernard, proposed that it was not just the pathogen but the person's susceptibility to the pathogen which led to illness.

This susceptibility, for why the person's own immune system could not combat the infection, has to do in part with the two other causes of illness, nutritional deficiencies and the body's total burden of toxins.

Pathogens are then the third primary cause of illness but in many cases, these pathogens are silent, meaning they don't produce acute symptoms such as a fever, but rather a host of chronic symptoms.

They are silent, low-grade and chronic, and normally don't show up on blood tests.

ONE ANALOGY OF DRUG SIDE-EFFECTS

Here we have a bowl, which represents the vessel of the human body, and will help to explain how we progress from health to illness in relation to chemical and drug toxins.

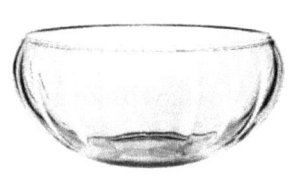

Imagine an empty bowl. This symbolically represents a state of health.

At birth the bowl is empty, yet over time, as we are exposed to environmental toxins and chemicals, our bowl slowly fills.

Even during this period of filling, we still feel well until the day our bowl becomes completely full and begins spilling over the edge.

This spilling over represents physical and mental symptoms, when the body's total burden of toxins is greater than the body's capacity to handle and excrete them.

These symptoms should warn us that something is wrong.

Unfortunately, this is the time when people visit their physician to be told that nothing appears abnormal on lab tests, with the blame placed on genetics, stress and age.

Most people then resort to over the counter medications or supplements to find relief.

This model explains why we may feel well up to a certain age and then begin to experience symptoms and a gradual decline in our health.

This is why, unless we address this accumulation of toxins, we shall never regain our health through drugs and natural remedies unless we engage purification therapies, or the emptying of the bowl.

This transition from health to symptoms is often subtle and can be triggered by what seems to be a slight insult, yet it is the accumulation of toxins over years and decades which is the underlying cause for this decline.

People with drug side-effects think it's their prescription, but it's not that simple, as this model explains.

People go to rehab with their bowl full of drug residues and chemical toxins.

No matter what you work through in sessions, no matter what breakthroughs you experience, you will never completely regain your physical and mental health until these residues are excreted, thus the benefits of NAD and other purification therapies.

There are two actions needed.

Stop Filling the Bowl

The 1st step is obvious, stop filling the bowl, stop being exposed to chemicals in our environment and the ingestion of toxins.

Anything that comes in contact with our skin is absorbed into the body.

What we inhale enters our bloodstream.

What we ingest enters both our bloodstream and lymph

system.

This reduction of exposure should be the basis of preventative medicine.

Empty the Bowl

The 2nd step is to empty the bowl. If we can drain the bowl then we can advance towards our original state of health and vitality.

You may remember what it felt like to have abundant energy, to run and play freely and to seldom feel exhausted.

I believe this abundant energy is still present in you and lies deep within.

This energy will never be accessed by a pill or supplement.

Your symptoms will never truly recede and your vitality will never resurface until you empty your bowl of toxic, poisonous residues.

There are several means of emptying the bowl which will be covered shortly.

Tipping the Scales

To add another perspective on the transition from health towards disease, I use the symbol of the Libra Scale to offer an explanation for the onset of symptoms.

When we are born the scale is tipped to one side, let's say all the way to the right.

This right side represents everything which promotes health including sunlight, fresh air, clean water, nutrient dense foods, a clean shelter, love, movement, creativity and a spiritual orientation to life.

The left side of the scale represents everything which is

harmful and destructive to life.

These insults include pollution, synthetic chemicals and drugs, chronic anxiety and stress, pathogens, a sense of isolation and many others.

As these insults are slowly loaded onto the left side, the scale begins to tip towards the left.

This represents the onset of physical and mental symptoms, when the body and mind are trying to communicate to us that something is wrong.

Chronic illness results when we do not put enough beneficial things on the right side and are not conscious of the insults being loaded onto the left.

When we advance from symptoms to a full blown chronic illness or disease, the scale has finally tipped all the way to the left.

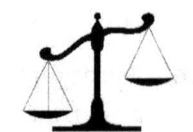

As you can see from this model, you can place all the vitamin supplements in the world on the right side, but they will never be enough to tip the scale all the way back to health.

To recover our health, we must simultaneously remove insults from the left, avoid them as best we can and load more benefits onto the right.

Feeding the right side of the scale seems pretty obvious; organic nutrient dense foods, purified water, movement, fresh air, sunshine, a sense of purpose and belonging, specific herbs and supplements, and many others.

When it comes to addressing the left side, this is bit more challenging.

Certainly the 1st step is to avoid what is harmful; pesticides, herbicides, chemicals, drugs, mold, common household cleaners, fluoride, heavy metals, artificial ingredients and sweeteners, pathogens and many others.

OK, so it's one thing to avoid these insults but it's another to remove them from the left side of the scale.

This is where various purification and intravenous therapies come in.

Purification Therapies for Recovery

This chapter covers therapies which assist detoxification pathways to rid the body of drug and chemical residues.

Toxins can be located in various tissues.

- Inside every cell of the body and brain
- Fat cells just under the skin
- In cells lining of the small intestines, called the Enteric Nervous System
- Lymph fluid

Before we begin to mobilize drug residues from inside our cells, it's important to move or drive the lymph system (clear the swamp).

Lymphatic Hydrotherapy

An old time naturopathic therapy with multiple benefits is the application of hot and cold compresses to the upper body, which was first introduced by two naturopathic physicians, Dr. Carroll and Dr. Harold Dick.

I was very fortunate to do part of my clinical internship with Dr. Dick.

When I arrived, I thought I'd just be an observer and pick up some clinical pearls along the way.

But he told me if I really wanted to understand the benefits of hydrotherapy, I'd have to experience it.

So twice a day, for three days, I also became his patient.

I tell you… after three days I felt amazing and decided to continue the therapy with the help of another student for seven more days after returning to school.

To say the least, I was impressed with how such a simple therapy could make such an immediate difference in my health and energy.

I will walk through each step of the treatment, to explain its benefits and why it is one of the best therapies to move and drain the lymph system and to support the body's innate ability to recovery.

The Procedure

You lie on your back on a massage table, undressed from the waist up, and covered with wool blankets from your neck to your feet.

The hydrotherapist pulls down the blankets to uncover your chest and abdomen, and a moist, thick hot compress is placed from just under the neck to the pubic bone, and to the sides of the chest and abdomen.

Once the compress is in place, blankets are adjusted to cover the hot compress and tucked tightly around the sides of the waist, chest and shoulders.

This heating compress remains for five minutes.

What is the body's response to this hot compress?

When heat is applied to the skin it causes a reddening, since fresh blood circulates into the small capillary blood vessels just under the skin.

But something else is going on here.

Over the entire body we have dermatomes which run in parallel lines along our skin. These dermatomes are rich in nerves which reflect, through the spinal column, deep into the body.

DERMATOMES

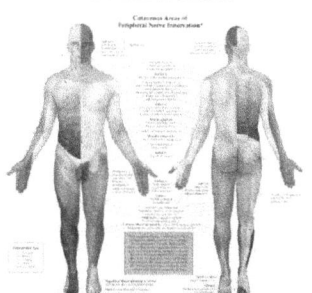

When a dermatome on the skin is heated, its corresponding internal organ(s), reacts in a similar way, with increased blood flow.

Heat placed on the skin, say at dermatomes 7, 8 and 9, will cause the dilation of blood vessels within the liver, with the corresponding increase in blood flow.

With the application of a hot compress over the chest and abdomen, all the underlying, internal organs will be filled with fresh blood causing increased oxygenation, increased delivery of nutrients and the removal of metabolic waste and toxins.

After five minutes, the hot compress is replaced by a cold compress, covering the same area of the chest and abdomen.

This cold compress remains for 10 minutes.

Now what is happening?

The body's _initial_ reaction to a cold compress is the opposite of a heating compress.

The blood vessels just under the skin constrict, driving blood into the core of the body. The skin will become blanched.

This same reaction is occurring to the internal organs as well since the dermatomes are sending a chilling or constricting message.

This is the initial, immediate reaction to cold (constriction) but then there's a <u>secondary</u> reaction.

The body will, after a few minutes, redirect blood to the skin to warm the cold compress.

As fresh warm blood is flowing to the skin, the same is happening to the internal organs.

This pumping action, of blood flowing back and forth to the skin and in and out of the organs, has many benefits including purification, increased oxygenation of tissues and the delivery of nutrients.

This alternating hot and cold also increases the activity of what's called the 'lymphatic pump' which transforms a lymphatic swamp into a river.

After the hot and cold compresses to the chest and abdomen, you turn onto your front and the same procedure, the 5-minute hot compress and the 10-minute cold compress, is repeated.

This therapy not only increases the flow of lymph but also improves digestive issues, blood sugar dysregulation and liver, gall bladder and kidney drainage.

Colon Hydrotherapy

The intestinal tract is one of the primary routes used by the body to expel drug residues and toxins, and must therefore be considered during purification.

When toxins are metabolized and filtered from the blood by the liver, they pass through the gall bladder on their way to the small intestines.

Once these toxins reach the gut they must then travel the entire length of the intestines, which is about 20 feet.

The faster we can move these toxins through the gut the less likely they will be absorbed back into the body.

During a purification program, as toxins are being released from cells, and the lymph is dumping them into the bloodstream, a person can feel unwell.

With colon hydrotherapy we can immediately reduce unpleasant detoxification symptoms.

The Procedure

We use a three-stage water filtration system.

The water is kept at body temperature and flows, at a very low pressure, through a sterile disposable speculum inserted into the rectum.

This is a closed system so there is no odor at all.

As the water slowly fills the colon, it works its way up the left side and then across the transverse colon.

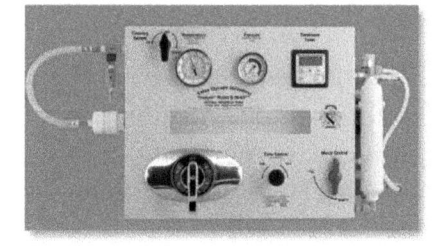

At some point the person feels the urge to evacuate.

The therapist opens a valve on the unit to allow all the fluid and fecal material from the colon to flow out the tubing and through an illuminated transparent glass tube in the machine.

Viewing what is passing through this tube may reveal undigested food, oil or fat globules, signs of Candida, and parasites.

Our colon hydrotherapist is fully trained and certified, with years of experience.

Saunas to the Rescue

I sincerely believe that if saunas were incorporated into our modern lifestyle, we would not be witnessing such a rapid decline in the health of our population.

Even the issues of pharmaceutical side-effects could be greatly improved since a lot of their residues are compartmentalized within fat cells just under our skin.

Getting drug and chemical residues out of this layer is easily accomplished through perspiration.

But a word of caution.

If heat penetrates too deeply, then some toxins released from fat cells will enter the body rather than out through the skin.

For this reason, we prefer the dry heat sauna over the infrared.

The Benefits of Sauna

For centuries saunas have been used by various cultures for purification, relaxation, spiritual rites and connecting with nature.

Yet how often do we sweat?

We go from our air-conditioned homes to our air-conditioned cars.

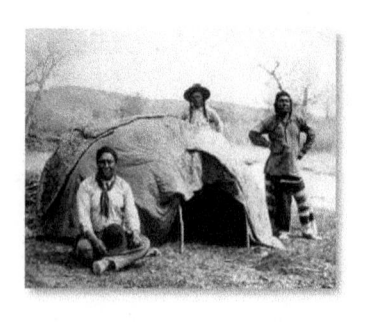

Many of us do not have a job that requires physical exertion and therefore we do not sweat.

We use antiperspirants and apply skin creams which leave residues that block the pores of our sweat glands.

So, saunas, if we are to improve our health, must become a part of our lifestyle.

The Sauna Experience

During the sauna experience you should feel completely relaxed. Therefore, perspiring during exercise will not be as beneficial compared with relaxing in a sauna.

We want blood to flow to our skin and not necessarily to our muscles.

This is key.

The more relaxed our muscles are the easier blood will flow from the body's core to the skin's surface.

This easier flow keeps the heart calm and maintains a lower heart rate and blood pressure.

Walk-in Dry Sauna

Our walk-in sauna is private unless you request another to join you.

There is plenty of room to lie down and to relax.

Next to our walk-in sauna is a shower.

If you remember the benefits of the alternating hot and cold compresses with Lymphatic Hydrotherapy, you will understand why we have located the shower so close to the sauna.

It's best to alternate between the hot sauna and a cold shower.

After working up a good sweat, and you sense the body would like a refreshing cool rinse, you exit the sauna and enter the shower.

Cold is another way to stimulate your mitochondria and even the release of stem cells.

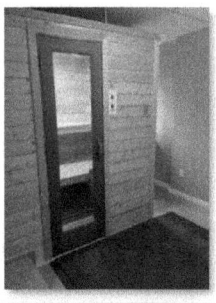

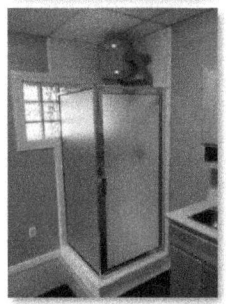

This cold rinse also prepares you for additional time in the sauna.

We recommend going back and forth between the sauna and the cold shower, always starting with the sauna and finishing with cold, and doing three cycles; hot/cold, hot/cold, and hot/cold.

The last cold can be warmer since it's important to remove oils from the skin using a chemical free soap.

The Bemer

Dr. Alfred Pischinger, MD (1899-1982) from Austria was the first scientist to describe the regulation of the Extracellular Matrix (ECM) and stated that health and disease are determined by the state or quality of this Matrix tissue, which includes the lymph system, or lymph fluid, and the fluid in the blood capillaries.

If this Matrix is clean and free of toxins, then the person will most likely remain healthy.

If it is unclean then the person will most likely become ill.

If the Matrix is running like a stream, then drug residues and toxins excreted by cells will more easily be swept away.

Let's talk about the capillaries, our smallest blood vessels, which are part of this Matrix.

As arteries become smaller (arterioles) and smaller, we finally come to the tiny capillaries through which red blood cells flow to deliver oxygen and to carry away waste.

Before each capillary is a tiny muscle called the pre-capillary sphincter.

If this muscle is constricted then red cells and blood flow are restricted.

What if we could help these tiny, pre-capillary muscles to relax?

Its relaxation would allow more red blood cells to flow through, thus delivering more oxygen to increase mitochondrial function, increased clearing of toxic residues and improved delivery of nutrients.

A German company was given the task of improving the health of the older population to reduce government spending on health care.

They developed the Bemer, which emits, what they call, specific micro-Tesla frequencies to relax these pre-capillary sphincters or muscles.

A Bemer treatment lasts eight-minutes, with a person lying on a full-length mat which emits these frequencies.

Besides the benefits mentioned, we use the Bemer before each IV therapy to enhance the delivery of nutrients to tissues.

Photon Sound Beam

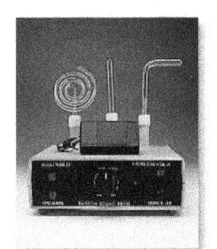

This unit emits high frequency waves, specifically those we call Rife frequencies and the multi-waves developed by George Lakhovsky.

These frequencies have proven to have many benefits including the disruption of pathogens, dissolving waste products such as biofilm, improved oxygenation of tissues, energizing cellular function and increasing lymphatic drainage.

It is a simple therapy but extremely effective and complements many of the therapies we offer.

LIST OF THERAPIES

Let's begin with an overview of various therapies which address the three primary causes of illness including the side-effects from pharmaceuticals.

Nutritional Deficiencies

- IV Vitamins, Minerals & Trace Minerals
- IV Alpha Lipoic Acid
- IV Glutathione Push
- IV BiOcean from France, rich in trace minerals
- IV Meyers Cocktail of Nutrients
- IV Plaquex for Cellular Membrane Repair

Environmental Toxins, Drug Residues & Biotoxins

- IV NAD
- IV Glutathione Push

General Detoxification (Emptying the Bowl)

- IV Alpha Lipoic Acid
- Lymphatic Hydrotherapy
- The Bemer for Clearing Lymph and the Matrix

- Colon Hydrotherapy
- Photon Sound Beam
- Walk-in Sauna with Cold Shower

Pathogens (bacteria, spirochetes, viruses & mold)
- IV Zotzmann 10-Pass Ozone Therapy
- IV UBI (Ultraviolet Blood Photonic Therapy)
- IV High Dose Vitamin C

Let's cover, in more detail, each of the above IV therapies.

Nutritional IVs

The Multivitamin, Mineral & Trace Mineral IV provides vitamin C, all the B-vitamins, various minerals like magnesium, calcium and potassium, and trace minerals such as zinc, manganese and selenium.

Alpha Lipoic Acid increases mitochondrial activity, repairs liver cells, and improves the detoxification ability of the liver. Lipoic acid is also an antioxidant and can potentiate the benefits of the IV vitamin C when administered afterwards.

Glutathione is an antioxidant, helps neutralize free radicals and improve the liver's ability to clear toxins from the blood. It is given as a push from a syringe directly into the vein.

BiOcean from France is deep ocean water, harvested and then processed through a sophisticated cold-filtration system leaving all minerals and trace minerals intact.

When the oceans retreated, our soil was rich in

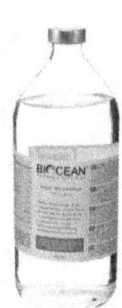

a plethora of trace minerals, but now, even our organic produce has become deficient.

Meyers Cocktail is a quick and simple means of delivering vitamin C, various minerals and B vitamins intravenously.

It is also referred to as a Meyers Push since these ingredients are drawn into a 60cc syringe, rather than a large IV bag, and slowly pushed over about 10 minutes.

Plaquex has been used for over 55 years in about one-quarter of the world's countries and was originally developed to resolve fatty embolus (plaque) during and after surgery.

In the 1990s its use shifted to complement IV EDTA chelation therapy, used for removing or dissolving hardened plaque from the walls of arteries.

Not only does Plaquex help repair the lining of arteries, it also improves the membranes surrounding all our cells.

A healthier cell membrane allows increased waste excretion and the uptake of vital nutrients.

Plaquex is designed to repair cell membranes that have been damaged by toxic substances, drugs, heavy metals, solvents and free radicals.

NAD IVs are the primary means of getting drug residues and other toxins to be excreted from inside every cell of the body and brain.

IVs for Pathogens

To discover if a person has issues with blood pathogens, we use both standard lab testing and looking at a tiny drop of a client's blood sandwiched between two pieces of glass (a microscope slide and a cover slip) under a dark-field microscope.

To address bacteria, including spirochetes, viruses and mold, we use the following IV therapies.

Zotzmann 10-Pass Hyperbaric Ozone Therapy

This treatment mimics the activity of our own white blood cells.

To kill pathogens, our white blood cells produce hydrogen peroxide, which is H_2O_2.

This molecule breaks down into H_2O (water) and a singlet oxygen. This single oxygen atom is what kills or oxidizes pathogens.

Ozone is O_3 and breaks down into O_2 and the same singlet oxygen.

Ozone and H_2O_2 reduce not only bacteria but mold as well, and cripple viruses to inhibit their replication.

Ozone has other health benefits including the increased oxygen carrying capacity of red blood cells and improving the function of mitochondria.

Our German Zotzmann machine allows us to treat about 2,000cc (2 liters) of a client's blood with ozone during a single session, which takes between one to two hours.

Most people have between four to five liters of blood, so we are treating about ½ the body's blood.

Sometimes, when a client's immune system is compromised, and their white blood cells are underactive, we will alternate between the Zotzmann and high dose vitamin C.

UBI or Bio-Photonic Therapy

This therapy has many benefits and is used to treat a wide range of issues.

It has been used by physicians for over 70 years, with over a million treatments given and not a single adverse reaction recorded.

Some proven benefits of this therapy are the following:

- Kills bacteria and molds in the blood
- Inhibits the replication of viruses
- Supercharges the immune system
- Improves microcirculation
- Oxygenates tissues
- Reduces inflammation
- Stimulates red blood cell production
- Increases the flexibility of red blood cells and therefore improves oxygen delivery to tissues

Most clinicians using UBI will typically treat about 60cc of blood at a time.

We have greatly modified this by using the UBI unit pictured above in conjunction with the Zotzmann.

A sterile IV line is attached to a butterfly, which is inserted into a client's vein.

This IV line has a special clear glass section which fits into the UBI unit, with the other end fitted to the 200cc sterile glass vacutainer connected to the Zotzmann machine.

The negative pressure, or vacuum, in this vacutainer draws

blood from the vein, through the IV line and into the sterile glass vacutainer, until we reach 200cc.

Then the Zotzmann delivers the ozone into the vacutainer, which is mixed with the blood.

Now we turn on our GHL 3000 12" ultraviolet unit while the ozonated blood is flowing back into the client's vein.

We repeat this same procedure once more.

So to clarify, 200cc of ozonated blood travels from the vacutainer through the UV unit only when it is flowing toward the vein, not when it is coming from the vein.

These two passes allow us to treat approximately 400cc of blood.

We have found this method far superior to treating just 60cc of blood.

At no time is the catheter or needle removed from the client's vein, and only disposable, sterile materials are used, so every step remains sterile.

High-Dose Vitamin C

Vitamin C is considered an anti-oxidant, but when doses upwards of 25 grams are administered intravenous, vitamin C causes an oxidative effect.

There is another reason for administering vitamin C.

Besides our white cells secreting hydrogen peroxide to reduce pathogens, white cells also do our housekeeping, by eating or phagocytizing debris and dead pathogens.

Please note that before administering any IV high-dose vitamin C, a blood test called G6PD is required.

Section III

Comprehensive Testing to Assess Underlying Causes

It would be overwhelming, and likely very boring, to explain the details of every lab we run for each client.

So we'll list each lab with some explanations of why.

LabCorp of America

Lipid Panel for Cholesterol and Other Fats

Fasting Glucose

HA1c (determines average blood glucose)

Liver or Hepatic Panel

CBC or Complete Blood Count for Red and White Blood Cells

Comprehensive Metabolic Panel (Too many components to mention)

Thyroid Hormones
- TSH
- T4
- Free T4
- Free T3

- TPO antibodies
- Thyroglobulin antibodies
- Reverse T3

Ferritin for men and post-menopausal women

C-Reactive Protein

Iron Panel

Urine analysis

G6PD (to know if someone can take high doses IV Vitamin C)

Viral Panel

Vitamin D

B12

DHA Laboratory

We run zinc, copper, histamine and the KPU.

The first two, looking for lows and highs, can often relate to psychological issues, with the third to know if someone is an under or over-methylator.

If they are under or over, then specific supplements are recommended according to the research of Dr. Bill Walsh.

The KPU is to know if the person requires high amounts of specific vitamins and minerals.

Cell Science Systems Lab

Now we are getting down to enzymes related to various pathways of detoxification at the cellular level.

This is a cheek swab to assess a person's genetic ability or inability to detoxify at the cellular level, and whether certain foods or specific nutrients should either be included or excluded.

This panel includes; MTHFR, MTR, MTRR, ACHY and COMT.

Labrix

We use Labrix for all our saliva hormone testing.

All hormones in the blood are either attached to a protein carrier, like being on a bus, or they are detached and referred to as free.

Only the free hormones are small enough to leave the bloodstream to enter lymph on their way to cells.

In general, and there are a few exceptions, blood lab tests for hormones measure the hormone bound to its protein carrier and the hormone that's free. This is referred to as the total amount of that hormone.

This is true for all the estrogens, progesterone and the adrenal hormone cortisol.

Testing these hormones through blood labs won't tell us how much of the hormone is free and available, which is what we want to know.

Therefore saliva, which is lymph, is the most accurate way to assess certain hormone levels.

Dark-field Microscope

Unless a person has full blown septicemia, which is a severe systemic bacterial infection, there isn't a blood test that will uncover a low-grade, silent, systemic bacterial infection.

Even the Lyme test has faults, with false negatives (*they actually do have Lyme but the lab results says they don't*) and false positives (*they don't have Lyme but the test says they do*).

We have found the most accurate means of determining if

someone has bacteria in their blood is to view a tiny drop of their blood under a dark-field microscope.

Dark-field simply means that when viewing this drop of blood under the microscope, the field, or background, is dark.

This is different from the bright-field microscope used in many hospitals.

When light passes through the microscope's condenser, through the slide and into the lens, any lipid or fat will be illuminated on the viewing monitor.

Bacteria, including spirochetes, have a lipid membrane, so they are easy to spot.

White blood cells are also visible, so we can see their size and activity, helping us to gain some knowledge about the health of a person's immune system.

Mold looks like scum or mucous with white specked highlights, or like a Christmas tree or a fern, also with these white specks.

This visual test is a great way to determine a baseline before any therapies, and to intermittently assess a client's progress.

Electrodermal Screening

Dr. Reinhold Voll, MD, developed a unit to measure the electrical resistance of acupuncture points.

All organs have a reflex point on the skin.

When a brass stylus or probe is placed directly on this point, if the corresponding organ or tissue is working well and healthy, the unit will give a reading of around 50.

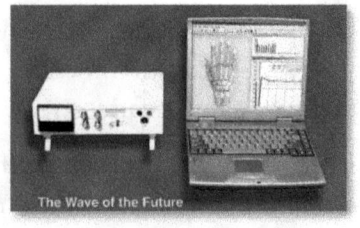

If the reading of this point is above 50, it indicates some degree of inflammation or possible infection, usually acute or sub-acute.

A reading of less than 50 indicates the corresponding organ or tissue is lowered in function and likely relates to a chronic condition.

As an example, if there is a low reading on the acupuncture point for the small intestines, it could mean a chronic intestinal bacterial or fungal overgrowth, a chronic food sensitivity or allergy, leaky gut, or even a parasitic infection.

To determine which it might be, we place various remedies into the circuit while rechecking the point to see which one corrects the low reading.

Therefore, this unit helps to know what the issue is and indicates the best approach to treatment.

This covers all the routine testing we do for every person.

Section IV

Summary & Highlights

Here are some highlights of what's been covered.

- The symptoms you associate with your prescription are due to many causes, and not just the medication.
- Most conditions are caused by nutritional deficiencies, environmental toxins including pharmaceuticals, and pathogens.
- These three causes lead to mitochondrial dysfunction.
- The primary aim is to increase mitochondrial function.
- The primary way to decrease physical and mental symptoms is to eliminate drug and toxic residues from within cells.
- Use various purification therapies to assist the body to excrete toxins.
- Use intravenous therapies to increase mitochondrial function, to improve nutrient levels, to support the immune system, to reduce pathogens and environmental toxins, and to improve the pathways of detoxification.
- Remember, you possess a miraculous innate physician which is dedicated to helping you to recover your health.

- Secure a mental attitude of respect and appreciation for this wisdom.
- This wisdom speaks to you through physical and mental symptoms, your conscience, intuition, instincts and common sense.
- It is your responsibility to support this wisdom and to learn its language.
- Realize that the vitality deep within your body and soul can never be restored through artificial means.
- Invest in your health, otherwise your savings and income will be consumed by medical expenses.

Section V

Becoming a Client

If you are interested in coming to our clinic, to take advantage of our services and therapies, this is how to proceed.

If you live close to our clinic then read the first section.

If you are from out of state, there are several things which must be done before your arrival. Go to the next section titled 'Long-Distance Clients'.

Clients in Utah

When you call our clinic and mention your interest in our program for treating side-effects from pharmaceuticals, Dr. Haskell will likely call you back the same day to answer your questions.

The next step is to forward our intake questionnaire to your email address.

Complete this questionnaire on your computer, save it and attach it to an email reply to AdvancingCare@gmail.com.

Dr. Haskell will review your answers and then contact you by phone to clarify your intent and to discuss the next step.

Most often, this next step is to come to our clinic for a fasting blood draw. This will cover the LabCorp and three of the DHA labs.

When you come for the blood draw, you will be given additional kits for collecting specimens at home.

- Saliva kit for various hormones
- Urine kit for checking KPU
- Cheek swab kit, checking MTHFR (*both heterozygous & homozygous*), MTR (*both heterozygous & homozygous*), MTRR (*heterozygous*), AHCY (*homozygous*) and COMT.

When all your lab results have arrived, your first appointment will be scheduled with Dr. Haskell and his assistant.

During this two-hour consultation with Dr. Haskell, the following will be covered;

- A detailed review of your symptoms
- A review and explanation of lab results
- Viewing a drop of your blood under a dark-field microscope
- Testing various acupuncture points on our EAV unit.
- Likely a brief physical exam
- Recommendations for various supplements to address underlying issues reflected in any of the lab reports
- Supplements to improve your pathways of detoxification
- Prioritization of the most important therapies to begin with
- Determining when you will be ready to start the ten days of IV NAD.

Dr. Haskell will likely recommend a number of nutritional IVs, and possibly to begin addressing blood pathogens or mold with the 10-pass Zotzmann or the UBI.

If appropriate, he will recommend scheduling a visit with our nutritionist and his daughter Justyn Manley, who is excellent when dealing with emotional issues and traumas.

You will come away with a very clear agenda, a timeline of how you will proceed along the path to recovery.

Each person is different in terms of how long it takes to do the entire program including the 10 NAD IVs.

Figure that from the time of your 1st consult to completing the 10 NAD IVs will be around three weeks to a month.

Everything is included in this program up to and including the last IV NAD.

- Dr. Haskell's review of your intake questionnaire
- All blood, urine, saliva and cheek swab genetic testing
- The initial two-hour consultation with Dr. Haskell
- Your visit with our nutritionist
- The initial one-hour consult with Justyn Manley plus three additional visits if needed
- A half-hour consultation mid-way through the program with Dr. Haskell
- A repeat of the dark-field microscope if progress needs to be assessed
- All supplements during the program, up until the last NAD IV
- All IVs which address the three primary causes of illness.
- Ten NAD IVs
- All purification therapies
    - Colon hydrotherapy

- Lymphatic hydrotherapy
- The Bemer
- Saunas
- Photon Sound Beam

At the time of this writing, the cost of the complete program is $10,000.

When you first arrive at our clinic for lab testing, we require a payment of $3,000.

When you arrive for your first consultation, we require a second payment of $3,000.

This covers everything; supplements, IVs and purification therapies, up to when you are ready for the 10 days of NAD.

When you are ready to begin the NAD, we require the final payment of $4,000.

PLEASE NOTE: VEIN ACCESS IS VERY IMPORTANT.

IF YOU HAVE HAD ISSUES WITH PREVIOUS BLOOD DRAWS THEN PLEASE LET US KNOW.

TO FACILITATE INTRAVENOUS THERAPIES, ESPECIALLY THE ZOTZMANN OR THE UBI WHICH REQUIRE FAIRLY LARGE BUTTERFLIES, YOU MAY NEED TO HAVE A PICC LINE OR PORT INSTALLED.

THE COST OF EITHER OF THESE IS NOT INCLUDED IN THE PRICE OF OUR PROGRAM.

Long Distance Clients

When you call our clinic and mention your interest in our program for treating side-effects from pharmaceuticals, Dr. Haskell will likely call you back the same day to answer your questions.

The next step is to forward our intake questionnaire to your email address.

Complete this questionnaire on your computer, save it and attach it to an email reply to AdvancingCare@gmail.com.

Dr. Haskell will review your answers and then contact you by phone to clarify your intent and to discuss the next step.

Most often, the next step is to mail lab requisitions and kits for checking your biochemistry and hormones.

Unless you are a resident of New York, Rhode Island or Connecticut, the process is very simple.

This is what you will receive by mail.

- A LabCorp requisition with instructions on how to locate one of their patient service centers and how to prepare for the blood draw.
- A DHA Lab kit, checking blood for zinc, copper and histamine
- Saliva test kit, checking various hormones
- A DHA Urine kit to check KPU (kryptopyrroles)
- Cheek swab, checking for MTHFR (both heterozygous & homozygous), MTR (both heterozygous & homozygous), MTRR (heterozygous), AHCY (homozygous) and COMT.

After you've been to LabCorp, we should have results within a few days. Other results may take 7-10 days.

If any results from LabCorp are a concern, you will be immediately called to schedule an appointment with Dr. Haskell.

Otherwise, if nothing stands out, we will wait until all lab results have been received before setting your first appointment, which will be long distance.

All lab results will be forwarded to you since it's very important for you to follow along during your consultation with Dr. Haskell.

There's a reason we begin with long-distance consultations, because you need to begin addressing issues before you arrive, to ensure the most benefits from all our therapies including the IV NAD.

During the first consultation, the following will be covered.

- A detailed review of your symptoms
- A review and explanation of your lab results
- Recommendations for various supplements or products to start before your arrival, which address underlying issues reflected in your lab reports and the symptoms you've discussed with Dr. Haskell
- Products will be suggested for improving your pathways of detoxification.
- You will be advised about some purification therapies you might be able to start before your arrival
- If Dr. Haskell suspects dental issues as being a cause for symptoms, this will be discussed.
- He will do his best to determine how soon you will likely be ready to come for all our therapies including the IVs of NAD.

You will come away from this initial long-distance consult with a very clear agenda, the steps you'll take along the path to recovery.

If Dr. Haskell suggests having a long-distance consultation

with our nutritionist, this will be scheduled.

Dr. Haskell will pass along his suggestions to our nutritionist, based upon your lab results and the symptoms he feels relate to your food choices.

He may also suggest a brief conversation with his daughter, Justyn Manley, who is an excellent therapist for emotional issues and traumas.

If you sense this is a good match, then subsequent visits will be arranged when you arrive at out clinic.

The day you arrive at our clinic, you will have a second visit with Dr. Haskell to review how you are doing, to view a drop of your blood under the dark-field microscope, a brief physical exam and the testing of acupuncture points.

An agenda for therapies will be discussed and scheduled.

Any additional supplements will be provided.

Most people coming from a long distance stay for three weeks. The first week is devoted to various purification therapies as well as nutritional, supportive and oxidative IVs.

The second and third weeks are for IV NAD, but other therapies will likely be included.

For your first week, it is best to schedule your first appointment on a Monday.

The first IV NAD always begins on a Monday as well, and administered every day for 10 days, usually skipping the weekend.

Everything is included in our program whether you stay for three or four weeks, up to and including the last IV NAD.

- Dr. Haskell's review of your intake questionnaire
- All blood, urine, saliva and genetic cheek swab testing

- The initial long-distance consultation with Dr. Haskell over the phone
- The consultation with our nutritionist
- The initial brief long-distance conversation with Justyn Manley and three other visits while you are here
- The second consultation with Dr. Haskell when you arrive
- A second consult with our nutritionist if you think you need one.
- All supplements recommended by Dr. Haskell during your initial consultation
- All supplements recommended by Dr. Haskell after your second consult here at our clinic
- All supplements up until your last IV NAD
- A repeat of the dark-field microscope if we need to assess progress
- All IVs listed in this book
- All IVs to reduce pathogens (Zotzmann and UBI)
- Ten NAD IVs
- All purification therapies
    - Colon hydrotherapy
    - Lymphatic hydrotherapy
    - The Bemer
    - Saunas
    - Photon Sound Beam

At the time of this writing, the cost of the complete program is $10,000, whether you come for two, three or four weeks to our clinic.

Before shipping any kits, we require a payment of $3,000. This covers labs, your initial consultation with Dr. Haskell and supplements.

When you arrive at our clinic, we require a payment of $3,000 which covers all the consultations, additional supplement, all IVs and purification therapies.

When you are ready to begin NAD, we require the final payment of $4,000.

We are an out-patient facility, but you will be sent our 'Hospitality Welcome Package' listing lodging, restaurants, entertainment and local, nature destinations.

Please feel free to reach out to us if you have any questions.

PLEASE NOTE: VEIN ACCESS IS VERY IMPORTANT.

IF YOU HAVE HAD ISSUES WITH PREVIOUS BLOOD DRAWS THEN PLEASE LET US KNOW.

TO FACILITATE INTRAVENOUS THERAPIES, ESPECIALLY THE ZOTZMANN OR THE UBI WHICH REQUIRE FAIRLY LARGE BUTTERFLIES, YOU MAY NEED TO HAVE A PICC LINE OR PORT INSTALLED.

THE COST OF EITHER OF THESE IS NOT INCLUDED IN THE PRICE OF OUR PROGRAM.

Contact Information

Clear Health Centers, LLC

3350 Highland Drive

Salt Lake City, Utah 84106

801.875.9292

AdvancingCare@gmail.com

https://ivnaddrugaddictions.com/